Prostate:

Navigating Prostate Issues as a Couple

Published by Jane N. Hughes Melbourne, Victoria

ISBN: 978-0-6488978-8-0

Edited by Anne Schmitt & Dr. Christopher Ringrose

Cover photo by Jane N. Hughes

Cover design by Jane N. Hughes

Interior design by Jane N. Hughes

Disclaimer:

The author of this book is not a medical doctor, and the information provided cannot be treated as a medical advice neither could it replace any doctor's advice. Any content provided in this book is for educational purposes only and should be treated as such. Any decision made regarding medical outcomes are solely the responsibility of the individual. The author shall not be reliable in respect of claims, damages or loss in connection to the information gained from this book. The names and characters used in this book are fictional.

Prostate:

Navigating Prostate Issues as a Couple

JANE N. HUGHES

Jane N. Hughes

Prostate:

Navigating Prostate Issues as a Couple

Are you, your husband or relative suffering from issues related to the prostate? Are you feeling lost and confused in the medical field with its million terminologies and different proposed procedures? If your answer is yes to these questions, then you are not alone.

There are many people just like you out there. These people might remain silent as they ponder this lonely and different world, but they can nevertheless feel overwhelmed.

This book is designed to explore the issues brought about by disorders of the prostate, the world of loneliness it creates, and the nightmares it can bring to some couples. While other family members might also be affected by diseases or issues of the prostate, the only other person who can fully understand what it means to have prostate issues is the partner of the affected person.

Their world becomes totally foreign to others, and without different kinds of support the illness can affect the institution of marriage and intimate partner relationships.

While this book is going to discuss issues related to the prostate gland it is not entirely a medical book. It is written to assist and support those who have no idea about these problems. The book also provides an overview of some of the issues men and their relatives go through due to prostate issues.

However, because of the topics covered, the book will use some medical terms where necessary as this is unavoidable. I will try to simplify the jargon as much as I can to enable those who cannot understand this field to find supportive information.

Prostate issues can bring pain and shame to those who suffer from conditions affecting this part of the anatomy. These affect their wives and partners mentally, physically, psychologically, emotionally and sometimes financially.

The issues of prostate disease also create rifts between friends and families by stigmatising the affected men, or downplaying the trauma created by having prostate problems.

Communities shy away from discussing anyting to do with reproductive organs and as a result this topic is regarded or viewed as a taboo. Since this is a 'no-go zone' topic, people suffer in silence as they feel they have no one to turn to when they are faced with health issues related to these parts of their bodies. There is also the fear that discussing any issues in relation to the body organs not 'deemed fit' might upset others, and even receive condemnation within some Communities.

As with every other part of the body, diseases can affect these reproductive organs, and there is no shame in discussing diseases of any part of your body. You are not offending anyone! Nevertheless, a lot of people suffering from diseases related to 'private parts' find themselves in mental anguish and alone.

I am not an expert since I am a non-fiction author; however, I am also a registered nurse who has taken short courses to further understand these problems. I have worked in different areas of health and have had exposure to what men and their partners go through after diagnosis of their prostate problem.

I have also been personally affected, having had a close relative who has gone through this journey; therefore, I feel it is worth putting this information down on paper. It is important to set it down, as little is written about how this medical condition can affect relationships.

Hopefully, some people can benefit from opening-up about their life journey – that is, losing their prostate and or living with prostate issues. A lot of men suffer in silence or look for groups where they can seek comfort and solace, while they try to learn about and understand what happens if they either lose their prostate or live with a prostate issue.

However, if you are not up to date with the internet or social media you might feel left out. Lack of information and isolation can take its toll in terms of loneliness that leads to depression, and that is where a book like this comes in handy.

Throughout my nursing journey, I have looked after men who have had prostatectomy (removal of the prostate), and dealt with one of my family members who went through the same procedure. I realised how this disease can create havoc for a man and his family, particularly the wife or partner.

I therefore developed an interest in why this disease can cause disharmony within the family set-up and have done extensive research on the topic; hence my desire to share with others going through this journey.

My experience has come from caring for three categories of men. First, the ones who entirely believe in their urologists and that their word is final.

Second, those who have no interest in knowing what happens with their bodies and have little understanding of what is ailing them.

Lastly, those who are on board with their condition and have gone a long way to do research and have a better understanding.
Where do you belong?

Understanding The Prostate Gland

Before I go any further let me define the prostate. It is a gland the size of a walnut located deep in the pelvis between the bladder and the penis. The prostate sits below the bladder and the urethra that runs through this walnut-sized organ from the bladder to the penis, allowing flow of urine.

The prostate has various functions: it enables urine to be transported from the bladder to the penis by the urethra; the prostate gland plays a role in hormone production; and it contributes to the production of some fluids contained in your semen. This fluid enables transportation of sperm during sex.

Therefore, if this small organ is enlarged or diseased, urine flow can be affected, attaining an erection can be challenging, and the issue of recreation and intimacy can be difficult.

However, not all men who have issues with the prostate suffer from weak erections. I would bet that not many men think about the importance of their prostate gland, particularly when they are young. Did you know where your prostate is located?

As men grow older their prostate gets larger; urine flow becomes very slow, and they tend to visit the toilet more often. Some men also feel as though they have not completely emptied their bladder. Most men might not notice they have prostate problems if their urine flow does not prompt them to see their doctors. Their sexual capacity may not change, and they might not have any symptoms at all.

Enlargement of the prostate can start earlier than one might expect; however, this process does not always end up being cancerous. A prostate can be enlarged but benign.

Due to lack of symptoms, most men do not visit their doctor for a check-up and life continues as normal until their urine trickles and toilet visits become frequent.

One urologist used to say as men got older three things got bigger - the nose, the ears and the prostate! (I am not quite sure about his rationale since I am not an expert, however it made me wonder why some men have big ears).

Despite the narrative about old men having prostate issues, it is worth pointing out that a considerable number of men as young as in their mid-forties find themselves suffering from prostate problems. It is therefore important to bear in mind that even young men can be affected, and that getting a check-up is vital in the case of any signs and symptoms.

An early detection of any abnormality allows it to be addressed sooner and offer a better chance of longer survival.

In this book, I will use different case studies to help you understand different procedures undertaken when men have prostate problems. I hope you gain some knowledge from this book even though it is not in any way giving direct advice on how to proceed with your diagnosis.

Consultation with your general practitioner and urologist is always the way to approach your health problems, so that you can get the right medical advice from professionals.

However, if you have a degree of understanding it might help you feel at ease while looking for ways to be treated. If you have some skills and knowledge concerning your prostate, that can help create a good relationship with doctors as they treat you or seek to educate you on your prostate issues.

Before discussing the first case study it is important to understand different terminology used when prostate tests are undertaken.

Prostate Specific Antigen (PSA)

The most common method used to detect any issues with the prostate is the Prostate Specific Antigen, also known as PSA. A PSA involves a blood sample which is taken to pathology for analysis. The blood test checks the level of protein produced by normal as well as malignant cells of the prostate gland and this is reported in nanograms per millilitre (ng/ml).

PSA therefore does not differentiate between normal and abnormal cells; it only provides a figure, and the higher the reading the more likely the possibility that something is not right. A rising PSA will prompt the doctor to send you for further investigations.

The following table shows the level readings of PSA:

PSA	Levels
Normal	0 to 4 ng/ml
Slightly elevated	4 to 10 ng/ml
Moderately elevated	10 to 20 ng/ml
Highly elevated	20 and above ng/ml

The lower the PSA the better for you, as it is an indication that your prostate might be free from cancer. On the other hand, a higher PSA might be an indication of cancer, although this is not always the case, as prostates can be enlarged without the presence of a cancer diagnosis.

Medical Assessment

Most doctors will undertake a review of your medical history, including that of your family, before they send you for further tests.

While taking your history they also do a physical examination to look out for any signs or symptoms. The first physical examination undertaken for prostate enlargement is the digital rectal examination (DRE).

This is where the doctor requests you to lie on your side and inserts his finger to feel whether your prostate is enlarged. While this examination can provide evidence of an enlarged prostate it is not conclusive and therefore your doctor can send you for further tests such as blood examination.

Digital examination is not painful; however, it can be uncomfortable for some men; generally, it takes less than a minute for the doctor to check out the prostate. If you have difficulty urinating, your doctor might also check out your penis and palpate your stomach as part of the physical examination.

Some men get very worried on hearing their prostate is enlarged – though as mentioned earlier, having a large prostate does not always mean that one has cancer. When visiting a doctor, shame is left at the door.

Other examinations the doctor might undertake before a concrete diagnosis could be a bone scan, magnetic resonance imaging (MRI), computerised tomography (CT scan) or prostate-specific membrane antigen (PSMA), and positron emission tomography (PET) scan, among others.

All these scans evaluate your prostate through a more detailed analysis. They can also detect whether you have cancer or not, and whether it is contained in the prostate, or has invaded the surrounding tissues.

Prostate Biopsy

This procedure involves removing some samples of your prostate tissue which are taken to a pathologist where they check for any evidence of cancer cells. To access the prostate for biopsy the urologist uses ultrasound as a guiding tool. A needle is inserted through the wall of the rectum, and the doctor can visualise the needle using Trans-Rectal Ultrasound (TRUS) as they collect quite a number of prostate tissues.

Alternatively, the urologist can go through the space between the testicles and the anus known as the perineum. This procedure also uses the ultrasound to take biopsy samples, and is called ultrasound guided trans-perineal prostate biopsy. The latter is said to have a lower risk of infection and rectal bleeding.

One of the advantages of this method is that it offers disinfection of the skin before access, hence reducing the risks of infection.

Therefore, when you visit your urologist and hear these words, ask them to educate you on the procedure and what they mean for you.

Due to the invasiveness of this procedure, the side effects of having prostate biopsy could be:

- Minimal bleeding from the rectum
- Presence of blood in stool, semen and urine in the weeks after the procedure
- Soreness on the site of the procedure (which eases as you recover).

Staging, Grading and Gleason Score

Staging, grading and Gleason score are commonly used terminologies in medicine when dealing with prostate cancers. In this case staging indicates where you stand in terms of your diagnosis, and it indicates the extent of your cancer.

The staging process might contain a combination of described symptoms, physical assessment, blood tests, pathology reports and imaging. Staging indicates whether cancer is contained within the prostate or has invaded the nearby organs, tissues, lymph nodes or bloodstream.

While I will not go deeply into these details you can understand that if cancer is contained within the prostate and no other indication of cancer elsewhere, it might be classified as stage one.

Grading indicates the aggressiveness of cancer, and is a system which uses a scale where 1 is regarded as a slow growing cancer whilst grade 5 as the highest and the most aggressive.

Where the score indicates slow growth, the doctors may use active surveillance over time with no urgency for invasive procedures unless the cells change over time.

The Gleason score also uses a scale with an indication that 6 and below is slow, while 10 is aggressive. Both grading and Gleason terminologies might go hand in hand; some doctors use the Gleason score while others will use the grading score.

Gleason score is divided into three groups according to numbers starting from 6, 7 and 8 to 10. The same principle applies-- if the grade is low doctors might decide to wait and observe through tests before they proceed with any major invasive operation or treatment.

Number 7 is made up of two numbers. Number 7 with a combination of 3+4 and 4+3 means that when 3 is the preceding number, cancer might be slow growing. However, when 4 is preceding cancer is in the middle range of aggressiveness. I am not sure how this calculation is arrived at.

Number 8 indicates an aggressive cancer but has a better outlook than 9 and 10. The aggressiveness is classified according to the presentation of the cancer cells from the biopsy samples.

The following table simplifies this discussion without causing too much confusion over the numbers:

Grading	Gleason score	Indication
Grade 1	6 and below	Slow growing
Grade 2	7 (3+4)	Slow to middle range aggression
Grade 3	7 (4+3)	Middle range aggression
Grade 4	8	Aggressive
Grade 5	9 and 10	Aggressive

While it is important to understand the dynamics of these readings, there is no need to dwell on them too much. All you need to know is: what stage is your cancer? Which group or Gleason score category are you in? And what are the next steps after your grading?

It is important to have an education session with your urologists to ensure that you understand different options available for your treatment.

Having the skills to deal with your body enables you to make the right and informed decision for your treatment.

Otherwise, you can be overwhelmed with all the information given to you all at once. If you do not understand the medical jargon at all, it is perfectly OK to ask your doctor to put the scenario in the simplest language possible to enable you to have a clear understanding of what is happening with your body.

There is no shame in discussing anything in relation to what ails you, as medical professionals deal with these cases all the time, and you should feel at ease and comfortable dealing with them.

A lot of people get confused with the use of these medical terminologies, and it can be difficult to explain to an already confused patient what each of them means. Therefore, it is important to take a close relative with you who can adopt the mindset to ask questions on your behalf and be able to explain to you later.

Before visiting the doctor, it is also a good idea to write down all the questions you would like answered.

Diagnosis of cancer can be devastating to a lot of people and families. It can create unsettling times within the family due to the uncertainty involved in having this disease.

However, taking your time before any treatment is important, since it provides you with the opportunity to settle down and think things through. If need be, getting a second opinion is also recommended so that you can make an informed decision on your disease management and the healing process.

Prostate Surveillance

Since you now have an understanding of the grading of prostate cancer, you will be aware that some people are put in a category of 'prostate surveillance', also known as watchful waiting.

This surveillance is recommended to those who have very slow growing cancer, contained in the prostate and the doctors might suggest continuing a watchful approach, rather than proceeding to any radical treatment.

The whole concept of prostate surveillance is to give the patient time to enjoy their life over a period of time while observing any prostate changes before undertaking any other radical prostate cancer treatments.

The surveillance does not mean that the doctors do nothing with your diagnosis. You will be required to have check-ups maybe every three months or so, depending on your doctor, and have checks on the levels of PSA. This does not mean that cancer is not growing -- it might be, but slowly. Some people manage to live with this prostate cancer for a long time, and in fact might die with it rather than of it.

The following case study looks at a middle-aged gentleman who found himself struggling to pass urine and visited the toilet many times at night.

His name is John.

John is a sixty-year-old man who is aging gracefully and undertakes some physical exercise to maintain a healthy lifestyle. He is also particular in his eating and drinking. John visited his doctor for a check-up to ensure everything was going alright.

The doctor recommended having a prostate blood test (PSA) as a normal routine. When the test came back it was a little bit elevated, but the doctor decided to send him for a biopsy to confirm that nothing sinister was happening with his prostate.

The results came back that the samples did not show signs of cancer and therefore the doctor recommended he have repeat tests after one year. The second PSA showed that the figures had elevated, and another biopsy was recommended which showed that John had a few samples which showed cancer, classifying it as Gleason 6.

Prostate surveillance was commenced, whereby John would be going for the blood tests 3 monthly, to keep an eye on his slow growing cancer. John continued to live his life as normal even though he knew this situation could change if there were signs that cancer was growing faster than expected.

John had no symptoms and needed no interventions. While John was lucky, this is not the case with everyone.

Benign Prostatic Hyperplasia (BPH) or Enlarged Prostate

This involves an enlarged prostate, but without any detection of cancer cells. The signs and symptoms of this condition are the same as those presented with all other prostate issues trickling of urine, urgency to pass water, being unable to fully empty your bladder and frequency of visits to the toilet.

Jake with enlarged prostate

The following case study represents a man who had (BPH) and the intervention undertaken.

Jake, a seventy-two-year-old man, is married with grown up children. He is completely healthy and only takes a few tablets for high blood pressure and cholesterol; apart from that he never thought he had any other issues with his body. Over time Jake realised his urine flow was very slow but thought it was part of the aging process and never went for check-up.

Finally, a visit to his General Practitioner prompted Jake to have a rectal examination to check the size of Jake's prostate. The GP informed Jake that his prostate felt big and therefore it was worth doing a blood test to see the level of his prostate specific antigen (PSA).

Jake's blood was taken and sent to pathology for analysis, and he was told to wait for the results. On the way home Jake had a million questions as to the outcome of his blood test. His thoughts were leaning towards his having a prostate cancer, and apart from his wife, Jake had no other person with whom to discuss his dilemma; anguish commenced.

After a week of waiting, the GP called Jake and said his PSA results was reading at one (1) which is very low, and the doctor did not think that Jake had prostate cancer. However, he sent Jake for further investigations - to undertake biopsy (samples of tissues taken from the prostate) just to make sure that Jake was fine.

The biopsy did not find any cancer cells in the many samples taken. Jake's case study shows that he has a non-cancerous enlarged prostate.

In this case Jake consulted his urologist who suggested having a procedure called Transurethral Rection of the Prostate (TURP) to improve his urine flow.

Transurethral Resection of the Prostate (TURP) (Shaving of the prostate).

This procedure does not involve any cutting of the body. The urologist removes part of the prostate through the penis guided by a camera through to the prostate and does the resection.

This procedure does not treat prostate cancer. It enables men to regain their urine flow and reduce the frequency and the time spent in the toilet trying to pass water.

While the procedure works, it does come with some side effects. TURP is used to treat Benign Prostatic Hyperplasia, which in layman's terminology is an enlarged prostate.

Side Effects of TURP

When any part of the body is not functioning well, and medical interventions are undertaken, some side effects might be experienced.

Thus, there are a few side effects associated with TURP procedure. While urine flow might be improved, some people might experience:

- **Urinary tract infection**: After TURP a catheter is inserted in place to facilitate healing, and some men may contract an infection. Some men might also have recurring urinary tract infections after the procedure.

- **Difficulty passing urine**: This is normally temporary, and mostly occurs in the first few days after the catheter is removed; so, a trial of void is undertaken to check bladder emptying with passing of urine.
  This indicates how much urine you pass and the residual in the bladder is checked using a bladder scanner.

- **Urinary incontinence** and the urge to go to the toilet urgently can persist, particularly immediately after TURP, and occasionally can be a long-term problem for some men.

- **Erectile dysfunction:** This can happen either temporarily or on a permanent basis. Some men experience difficulty maintaining an erection after this procedure. If erectile dysfunction existed before the procedure, it might never recover.

- **Dry orgasm:** Remember the prostate contains fluid which transports semen; since TURP removes part of it, men cannot ejaculate like they normally do. That does not mean they do not experience orgasm; however, the experience may feel different from normal as semen goes back to the bladder rather than coming out from the penis.

- **Infertility:** Your fertility might be affected after TURP.

- **Retreatment:** Like every procedure, TURP might not fix the targeted issue. In this case there will be a need for retreatment if symptoms do not improve, or if they return over time. TURP may cause stricture (narrowing of the urethra) and this can cause difficulty passing urine.

Holmium Laser Enucleation of Prostate (HoLEP)

There is another option for having a prostate 'shaved' to enable easy passage of urine, known as Holmium Laser Enucleation of Prostate (HoLEP).

This procedure uses laser to treat the obstruction of urine flow due to an enlarged prostate (BPH). HoLEP enables urologists to remove tissues of the prostate without having to make any incisions on the body and offers better outcomes for the patient in terms of reducing the risks of bleeding.

However, the side effects of HoLEP can be leakage of urine after the procedure, and retrograde ejaculation (going back to the bladder, as mentioned above).

HoLEP procedure does not interfere with erectile function of the prostate. Therefore, this procedure enables the patient to continue living their normal lives.

There are risks in undertaking any procedure, and it depends on where you live, but if you are in the western world most medical facilities have programs and support in place to improve the lives of men undergoing these side effects. There is no point shying away from issues and suffering in silence. Utilising whatever is available to improve your mental, emotional and physical health is important to living a fulfilling life.

Can you imagine how life can change in a blink of an eye? One day you are enjoying your life and think that dripping of urine is the normal thing at your age, and the next thing a trip to the doctor tells you a different story.

This is the time you need support: somebody you can talk to, maybe a person who has undergone this procedure or journey and can relate to your own. Your family's support is important, and yes, most men do not want to be seen as weak, but there is nothing wrong with reaching out and talking about what is happening in your life.

Living in isolation creates other issues. You risk suffering from depression. It is important to seek professional advice and counselling if this is a problem for you. Over my early years as a nurse, I never realised how important a role the prostate played in males' daily life.

Working with men who have undergone different prostate procedures has changed my thinking dramatically, as I realised that the prostate is hugely important to a man, and that once it is gone men can think their manhood itself is completely absent.

However, you are not alone; there are many men out there who have lost their prostate and go on to live a fulfilling and satisfying life. You need to develop a positive attitude to enable you to move on and live fully and well.

Prostate Cancer

It is impossible not to be shocked when doctors mention the 'big C' as a diagnosis. However, not all cancers are aggressive, and even then, if yours is picked up early the chances of surviving are better if the condition is well managed. Prostate cancer is a blanket name for a number of different cancers, and the most common cancer of the prostate is called adenocarcinoma.

There are other types of prostate cancer, but they are very rare and can be very aggressive with a poor prognosis.

These are: -

- Small cell carcinomas
- Neuroendocrine tumours
- Sarcomas.

If you are diagnosed with adenocarcinoma of the prostate, which is the most common, There are a few treatment options out there.

Your work is to undertake all the research, discuss all the options available with your doctors and decide what will suit you best, for your own satisfaction or needs.

This will enable you to live comfortably knowing that the decisions you made about your treatment came from you with good advice, and that you were not compelled to make them.

Keith - Prostate Gleason Score 8

The next case study concerns a young man by the name of Keith who found himself suffering from prostate cancer.

Keith was a forty-five-year-old man, young at heart and physically active. He was married to Ann and they had three beautiful children. The children were in their teens, and Keith and Ann were just enjoying their lives now that they were not so busy. The teens were a little more independent and they could look after themselves to a point.

Both Keith and Ann were discovering the freedom they had before parenthood, and their marriage was strong. However, Keith noted that even though he did not have any obvious symptoms, his urine flow was not as strong as it used to be when he was a little bit younger.

Keith's interest in sex had declined, as the issue of waking up frequently to go to the toilet was disturbing him and making him tired. Even though he openly communicated to his wife about almost everything, they did not discuss their sexual life, and therefore he was not too keen to raise this issue with Ann.

During his routine check-up with the doctor, he mentioned that his urine flow had reduced, and the General Practitioner decided to carry out the rectal examination. Keith's prostate was enlarged. The GP also suggested they should arrange a PSA blood test and wait for the results.

After a week of waiting, that dreaded phone call came through to tell Keith that his PSA was very high, and more investigations were needed to find out whether his prostate had cancerous cells.

This news hit Keith hard, and he discussed the situation with Ann; together, they decided to follow up with the doctor's advice. The next step was to undergo a biopsy and taken to pathology for analysis. The biopsy was done as an outpatient appointment, where Keith was put under anaesthesia while the urologist took some tissues. A scan was also done.

The results came back showing that some tissue samples from the biopsy had cancer cells and graded it at Gleason score 8. Keith was informed that his cancer was contained within the prostate and this was confirmed by a scan.

The urologist recommended undertaking radical robotic prostatectomy. They had a good talk with Keith and re-assured him that there was life after prostatectomy and that he was going to try and save his nerve bundles so that he could resume intimacy with Ann.

Keith agreed to go ahead with the prostatectomy. However, mentally Keith was agonising, and the lack of sleep due to the bad news of hearing the 'C word' was devastating. Keith was still young and had a lot of his life ahead of him, and this was his prime time where he was enjoying his marriage.

Keith never thought young men his age could be affected by prostate cancer and so his research to find out what this prostatectomy involved commenced.

Keith's case study helps us understand that prostate issues are not just restricted to older men, even though there is that perception within society. This perception needs to change to enable men to secure better advocacy for their health.

What is prostatectomy?

Prostatectomy is the removal of the prostate gland -- remember that only men have this organ. Prostatectomy might be performed in the conventional way, whereby the surgeon makes an incision on the lower abdomen and manually removes the prostate.

Another way of surgically removing the prostate is by using the robot, also known as Robotic Assisted Radical Prostatectomy (RARP).

The surgeon uses a robot (key-hole surgery) to operate on you when he removes the prostate and attaches the urethra to the bladder. After this procedure is done, he manually removes the detached prostate and closes the incision sites.

The incision can be located at the belly button or below the lower abdomen; this depends on the operating urologist. At times, even with the availability of a robot, your surgeon might decide to use the conventional method for one reason or another.

Benefits of Robotic Prostatectomy

- Minimal invasion
- Minimal blood loss
- Fast recovery
- Better erectile function (if some nerves are spared, and no pre-surgical erectile dysfunction)
- Reduced chances of infection
- Shorter stay in hospital.

Having your prostate removed is a huge decision and it needs to be made in consultation with a multidisciplinary team. It is also important to discuss with your partner the way forward after prostatectomy, since there may be lifestyle changes due to the side effects associated with this procedure.

The removal of the prostate affects both you and your partner. More about this will be discussed later. Keith's wife Ann had to support him throughout the treatment and after, since Ann's life would also be affected.

One of the side effects of prostatectomy is erectile dysfunction. It takes a lot of patience and learning to enable couples to manage their new lives. While couples can be strong and learn how to adapt to their new lifestyle, this procedure has also contributed to the break-up of marriages. Therefore, counselling and talking to other people who have undergone it might support you and prevent much mental anguish.

Conventional Prostatectomy

Even though conventional prostatectomy is n o longer so popular, some urologist prefers to undertake this procedure. Conventional prostatectomy is an open surgery where an incision is made on your lower abdomen that enables the urologist to manually resect and remove the prostate.

Sometimes your geographical location and logistics of travel might contribute to the decision to perform a conventional prostatectomy. If there is no robot in your local hospital, the urologist will open your abdomen to remove the prostate.

The use of conventional surgery means that it takes longer to recover from this procedure. There are also higher risks associated with bleeding and infection. Cosmetically, the scar of the surgery can be ugly to look at, though few patients would not be overly concerned about the scar if the cancer had been dealt with.

Other Prostate Cancer Treatments

There are other types of treatment available for prostate cancer, and you need to undertake enough research to evaluate which treatment fits you and your diagnosis. Consultation with your doctors also helps you make a well-informed decision that is right for you.

After the decision is made, you need to live positively with your choice of treatment. Remember that since there is no going back, you cannot afford to regret your choice.

Brachytherapy

You might hear this word for the first time if you have been diagnosed with prostate cancer. Brachytherapy is an internal radiation where seeds containing radiation sources are placed near the tumour -- in this case within the prostate gland.

This is a minimally invasive procedure, and it ensures that the seeds are placed in the right area of the gland. A plan is put in place with a team of professionals involved in designing the treatment plan. This includes a radiation oncologist and the physics team. Who would ever have thought physics would be important in such cases?

I am not going into further explanation here about how the procedure is undertaken; if you opt for this treatment, ensure you learn from your oncologist what it involves. The aim of these radiation sources in the seeds is to kill the cancer cells without causing much damage to healthy surrounding tissues. There are two types of brachytherapy treatment: high dose and low dose rate.

High dose rate brachytherapy delivers radioactive sources in the prostate at a high dose of radiation for a short time before the sources are removed. It includes inserting thin tubes into the prostate gland before a source of radiation is passed through the tubes into the prostate for a few minutes to destroy the cancer cells. The radiation source is then removed. Since the radiation is put directly into the prostate, the healthy surrounding tissues receive a smaller dose of radiation.

Sometimes repeated treatment may be undertaken to achieve the optimal goal.

Low dose rate brachytherapy is a more protracted type of treatment where the aim is to insert the radioactive seeds for a longer term or on a permanent basis. This allows the radiation to be slowly released to the tumour in smaller doses over a longer duration.

Like many procedures undertaken brachytherapy has its own side effects. The side effects are not dissimilar to those of prostatectomy:

- Urgent needs to urinate at the onset of the treatment but eases after some time
- Erectile dysfunction
- Pain when urinating
- Bleeding from the rectum
- Urgency in bowel movements and more frequency, sometimes resulting in diarrhoea
- Blood in the urine or faeces.

Not everyone experiences the same side effects; it all depends on how your body reacts to different treatments.

Radiation (External Beam Radiation Therapy)

This involves the delivery of high external radiation beams to the affected area with the aim of destroying and killing cancer cells which grow and divide.

The treatment can be administered as a first line treatment of low-grade prostate cancer, which is confined to the prostate. It can be combined with other treatments (such as hormone therapy), to treat a more serious prostate cancer, a recurring cancer or advanced cancers, as a way of palliative comfort and pain relief.

The radiation treatment itself takes very few minutes, however preparation for the procedure takes quite a bit of time. The procedure is painless since it feels like having an X-ray. Earlier preparation is required to achieve the intended objective such as drinking water to fill up the bladder before the procedure and an enema for bowel preparation.

There are different types of radiation treatment including an oral drug targeting the tumour. EBRT is just one of these.

Like every other prostate treatment, radiation comes with some of the side effects discussed earlier; in addition, some patients might experience bowel problems such as diarrhoea. It is important to follow the instructions given by your radiologists before the procedure.

Hormone Therapy for Prostate Cancer

Since this book aims to provide a general understanding of the issues associated with prostate disease, I will not discuss in depth the medical terms in relation to these hormonal therapies; rather I will give a quick overview of what they are and what they do. Remember before commencing any treatment to consult widely until you attain an understanding and satisfaction.

Testes produce male hormones (androgens) known as testosterone, and this is converted to dihydrotestosterone (DHT) in the prostate; these hormones make one display the characteristics of a man. It is not necessary to remember all these terminologies; all you need to know is that to exist as a man you must have the above-mentioned hormones. Androgen can also stimulate prostate cancer cells to grow.

Without going more deeply into the science of the roles of these hormones, we can note that the work of hormone therapy is to suppress the levels of male hormones (androgens) in order to slow the growth of prostate cancer cells. In this case different methods are used to reduce or deplete the work of androgens. These methods may be surgically enforced, or drug related.

Orchidectomy is a general term to refer to a surgical procedure to remove the testicles. For the treatment of prostate cancer simple orchidectomy is performed where the testicles are removed, and prosthetic ones used to replace them. In other words, removal of testicles enables castration by removing the testicles where androgens are made; this stops prostate cancers from growing or makes them decrease over time.

Some men find this procedure very confronting and might not agree to it, due to fears that they might lose their manhood. Some might prefer to take low dose medication to reduce the hormone production, hence shrinking the testes or diminishing their work. This is referred to as medical castration as over time the testicles become very small in size.

These hormone treatments are administered to those cancers which have grown beyond the prostate gland and when there may be no other way of managing them. At other times, they may be administered as a precaution to ensure that the prostate has shrunk in size to enable other treatment to take place.

With these treatments the side effects might be different to all other prostate related treatments, such as:

- Decreased desire for sex (low libido)
- Depression
- Hot flushes
- Shrinkage of testicles and penis
- Erectile dysfunction
- Osteoporosis (brittle bones which break easily).

Nobody can underestimate the anguish this disease causes men, and I had a relative who preferred not to take hormone medication since his manhood was going to be affected.

One might regard it as foolish to think that way, since life amounts to more than a castration; but it is not unusual for people to prefer the consequences caused by cancer rather than lose their manhood. Sad to say, we lost that relative to prostate cancer since no amount of counselling was going to change his mind.

Chemotherapy

Chemotherapy can also be recommended as a treatment, and this depends on the treating urologist. Chemotherapy is used for advanced prostate cancers with distant metastasis (grown out of the prostate). This type of treatment has been shown to extend and improve quality of life for many patients. There are different chemotherapy drugs which are used to manage advanced prostate cancer. The obvious side effects of chemotherapy are well known.

Considering all the different treatments discussed in this book, you can understand why this is best seen as a couple's disease, as the side effects will affect your relationship in one way or another.

The following discussion focuses on dealing with incontinence of urine after prostate treatments.

Urine Incontinence

You can imagine having a great fulfilling lifestyle that just disappears within a short time after seeking treatment. It can be mentally draining for you and your family. I guess when women reflect back after being confronted by the effects of this disease. They might regret the times they declined to be intimate with their husbands or partners.

Remember that the prostate sits under the bladder and once it is removed there is no buffer to stop urine from flowing freely. To most men undergoing surgery this could be a positive thing as they suffered with urine dripping before the removal of their prostate. Therefore, when they can pass water without any issues there is an element of satisfaction.

The only problem of passing urine like a baby is that one must learn how to control it from flowing anyhow and anytime. This is where pelvic floor exercises play a role in getting your life back to near normal. Before any procedure is undertaken, you are advised to visit a pelvic floor physiotherapist to support and guide you through Kegels exercises.

These exercises strengthen your pelvic floor muscles so that after the prostate treatment you can control your urine if the right muscles are used. Kegel exercises continue to be undertaken even after undergoing the prostate treatment, to achieve an optimal outcome and enhance your wellbeing. They need to become a lifelong exercise if incontinence is to be under control.

Age also matters as to how much exercise you can undertake. If you are young and healthy it is easier to undertake pelvic exercises, and this contributes to better control of urine incontinence. The reference to age does not mean that if you are older, you are not able to undertake the exercises; there are some men out there who are older and still able to achieve control of urine. Each person is different and therefore some people are quicker to control their urine than others.

Some men manage to fully control incontinence, while there is a percentage who do not manage to do so well. Whichever category you fall into, you should have the will power to continue to strive to undertake pelvic floor exercises to reduce urine leakage to a point where a small amount can be absorbed using a pad.

Urine incontinence can be a deterrent for socialising or wanting to go out, and this can impact your daily life. Having a positive outlook on this situation is the best approach – as in learning a new skill -- teach your mind that you are a new person. Despite how difficult it seems, you will conquer this problem and learn how to live with it. After a few weeks of using big pads and undertaking Kegel exercises, you will graduate to a medium pad, then a smaller pad and eventually no pads at all.

There are a lot of new pads available which enable people to feel at ease going out to interact with others without feeling that they are smelling of urine. One thing you must remember is that there are many people who wear pads all the time, and you would never know or recognise them within the community. There is a joke which goes "I laughed until I wet myself"! When you have had a prostatectomy, this becomes a reality and not a joke anymore.

Catheter After Prostatectomy

After the removal of the prostate or some certain treatments, an indwelling catheter is put in place. This is a plastic tube put in after the operation and it is secured with an inflated balloon to hold it in place, to facilitate healing. This catheter can be left in place between seven and ten days, even though at times it might be in longer if issues arise.

Once the catheter is out, urine has nothing to stop it from flowing. During the operation the internal sphincter which control the flow of urine is close to the prostate and therefore is resected and this explains why you are unable to control urine and flows freely.

Having a catheter in place is very uncomfortable, and the urge to go to the toilet is ongoing since you have a foreign body in the bladder. In this case there are high risks of developing urinary tract infections and this can delay the healing process as well as delaying the removal of the catheter.

At times, men who develop a urinary tract infection will have an indwelling catheter for more than a week depending on their response to treatment. Nobody would wish this to happen, but it is one of the possibilities, and if it does occur the best thing to do as a patient is to look after that catheter.

Ensure that your hands are washed before and after touching the area involved. Follow your doctor's instructions and medications as required.

During the time you have a catheter in place, sometimes urine can bypass the catheter and leak around it; in this case a big pad is put on to ensure that urine is absorbed. It takes patience to go through the catheter phase. Be kind to yourself and give the body time to sort itself out.

Attached to the catheter is the urine bag that receives your urine, and for the first few days a large urine bag is used. Then the large bag is only used at night, and during the day you can use a small bag which is attached to your leg.

Dealing With Your Wife or Partner While Experiencing Incontinence

For better and for worse you still love your husband/partner, even through difficult times, and hope to get through this together. However, this period of incontinence can be demoralising, and your partner may feel frustrated at times if things do not progress in the right direction.

As for those who share the same bed, this phase can be disturbing for the other person. Support is vital but giving the other person space to reflect and be able to cope is also important. Some people prefer to go on sharing a bed, even in their initial time of healing. Others prefer to use a spare room for these first few weeks for privacy, and to avoid sleep disruption. Whichever way you find better, do it, so you are both comfortable with each other.

During the first few weeks, most men find long pants uncomfortable, so choose loose track pants or loose shorts which can provide comfort. Walking around the house or garden is good exercise; it helps to avoid blood clots from forming and facilitates quick healing.

Since the prostate provides a cushion between the pelvic bones and the bladder, once it is gone there is nothing between, so sitting down can be uncomfortable - look for a soft or doughnut cushion to prevent pain and discomfort if necessary. It's all right to use the medications given to control pain. While it is difficult to eliminate pain, if it's put under control, you can achieve better mental well-being.

Male Sling to Control Post Prostate Incontinence

If after some time you cannot seem to control the flow of your urine, there are some treatments which can reduce incontinence, such as a male sling.

Since incontinence can be debilitating and lead to lack of desire to do anything, some men prefer to seek other means to control their urinary incontinence. When you lose your prostate, you also lose the internal urethral sphincter and weaken the external one which enables the muscle to contract and control urine.

There are different types of procedures men can acquire if their incontinence does not improve over time. That is to say that, if more pads are used and there is no sign of improvement five years after prostatectomy then there is a good indication that the pelvic floor exercises did not yield much in achieving contraction of muscles.

A male sling is a synthetic mesh like tape inserted and positioned around part of the urethral bulb. The purpose of this sling is to slightly compress the urethra and position it close to the area of urethral sphincter. This type of procedure is designed for men with mild to moderate urinary incontinence.

The sling is inserted through an incision on the perinium (between the scrotum and the anus) and it is not a major operation, generally resulting in quick recovery. The procedure is done as an outpatient and you go home the same day. A catheter is put in place for two to three days but this depends on the operating surgeon.

Like every procedure some of the side effects of male sling could be:

- Inability to urinate or retention of urine which might require reinsertion of catheter
- Bleeding or infection
- Erosion -- but this is rare
- Recurrent leakage of urine.

The outcome of the sling insertion is generally positive, as some men report a curing of incontinence and have their lives back. Some have an improvement in their incontinence and others might look at other procedures such as artificial urinary sphincter to improve their situation.

Artificial Urinary Sphincters

The artificial urinary sphincter comes in three components: a ring-like cuff, a balloon filled with fluid and a pump. The cuff is placed around the urethra and enables the bladder to be shut until it is time for you to urinate. The cuff acts as a valve.

The balloon holds the fluid to ensure the cuff is always closed when no need to urinate.

The pump is placed under your skin on the scrotum, and it is used by pressing the pump when you feel the urge to visit the bathroom. The pump deflates the sphincter so that urine can flow out of your bladder. You can mechanically control your bladder, and this provides you with great freedom.

The other type of artificial urinary sphincter comes with two components: a cuff and a pump. Again, the cuff is placed around the urethra and the pump in the scrotum. It seems that this type of sling is not commonly used, since there is very little information concerning its use.

However, bear in mind that there is no complete guarantee that the sphincter will fix your problems even though the research shows that ninety percent of patients can control their urine using it. Unless you are unlucky enough to be in the ten percent, the ninety percent is a positive indicator.

The urinary sphincter is inserted in the operating theatre under anaesthesia and the patient stays in the hospital for two days for observations before being discharged home.

Sex After Prostate Treatment

Almost all prostate treatments and procedures deplete the work of the prostate by disabling sexual desires and erectile functions. Sex is an important part of marriage and having issues with the prostate has led to divorce in some cases. While a man is undergoing radiation the desire to have intimacy might not change in the early days of treatment but over time this desire may wane, and impotence may occur.

Some couples are very open with each other about their sexual life, but others prefer to keep it quiet. However, when you have problems with the prostate and are faced with the side effects brought by the treatment this may change. Many couples are forced to face the reality and discuss their next move after prostate treatment and procedures.

This honest discussion can be facilitated by your urologist or urology nurse who deals with sex education.

For some men, life completely changes after prostate treatment, but some few men are lucky enough to regain their sexual desire and actions a few months or years after treatment.

If you are younger and the nerve bundles of the prostate were saved through the operation, there is a high chance that you will recover and regain your sexual life. It is not a guarantee but a possibility. The older you are the harder it becomes to be sexually active, since in general desire reduces with age.

There are drugs and other tools which are designed to assist couples in regaining their sexual life, even though it may never be the same as before. The drugs might be used with a combination of other tools such as a pump if you have had prostatectomy. Again, it can be a long road to recovering your sexual activity, if it does ever recover. Who ever thought your sexual life would be a discussion with a third party?

Regaining sexual activity is also a mindset, and with a lot of work, positive thinking and support you may achieve your long-lost glory. But it is the case that some men may never regain their sexual life after these prostate procedures.

Penis Pump (Vacuum Erection Device)

After prostatectomy it is important to keep your penis healthy and promote blood flow to this organ. Therefore, a penis pump is one of the tools used to promote a healthy penis and to rehabilitate it to start working again.

The pump is an acrylic cylinder which is placed around the penis, with a ring to put at the base of the penis to avoid any escape of air. You gently pump the cylinder and the vacuum that is created enables the blood to flow into the penis making it rigid and erect.

This might only happen when the vacuum is pumped and even if you gain erections, they might not be enough for sexual penetration; however, it does encourage blood circulation.

The use of a penis pump also promotes the healing of nerves, as the blood carries nutrients healthy for your body -- in this case the penis. After surgery you lose some of the length of your penis and using the pump encourages the preservation of penis length.

Some men find it difficult to use the pump; they might say they are uncomfortable, or they cannot see any results. Despite the challenges, even when you do not get an erection, if the penis is healthy there is hope of restoring some intimacy. At times men completely give up and decide their lives are better off without using something like a pump.

This is all right if men are single, but when there is a woman or a partner involved, it is important to have consensus that both can survive without having penetrative sex. There are other ways couples can have intimacy and gain the same satisfaction; but if you are one who enjoys penetrative sex then frustrations can occur in relationships.

Oral Tablets

Erectile dysfunction is considered a condition just like any other, the only difference here being that you can decide whether you would like to be treated or not. You can live without being treated and that should not affect your life in general. However, where relationships are involved proper consultations and communication with your wife/partner are important so that both of you can make decisions based on your interests.

Oral tablets for erectile dysfunction are provided for intimate reasons, and even though this is important, they can also encourage the penis to be healthy by allowing blood to be pumped to this organ. Nobody would like to have a penis which is flaccid and not healthy.

There are a few of these drugs out there in the market and they must be prescribed by a qualified doctor. These medications are Sildenafil, Vardenfil, Tadalafil and Avanafil. They are vasodilators, meaning they widen the vessels to allow more blood to get to the penis.

Though these drugs are used to treat erectile dysfunction they are also used for other conditions such as pulmonary hypertension.

Remember that with every treatment there might be side effects associated with using such drugs.

The most commonly felt side effects of using oral erectile dysfunction medications are:

- headache
- body ache and pains
- flushes
- dizziness
- digestive problems (diarrhoea).

Where oral tablets do not provide you with a satisfactory result, there are other options offered by your doctor to address the issue of erectile dysfunction. These are injectable medications which are directly administrated to your penis.

Some medications can block others from working – for example, if you are suffering from hypertension and heart related diseases.

Medications provided to control hypertension or heart-related diseases can create erection dysfunction for some people. In this case it is important to check with your doctor regarding the safety of certain combinations of medications.

Penis Injections

Most men are protective of their penis, and treat it with the due diligence and tenderness it deserves. Anything like a sharp object going near this organ would be a nightmare for a man, and they might look at you and think you have lost your mind for suggesting a penis injection.

However, this is very practical – sometimes men who have lost their prostate may end up using penis injections to achieve their erections. There are also other conditions such as diabetes, heart conditions and high blood pressure which can affect a man's performance, and hence, they too tend to betreated using penile injections.

While injections are there to enable men to help live their lives fully, they are not a guarantee. Some men still fail to achieve their intended goal of enjoying penetrative sex and intimacy, even after having an injection.

Types of Injections

Caverject and Trimix are the most commonly used drugs to improve erectile dysfunction. Caverject is the second line of treatment where oral medications have failed to produce any results. It contains prostaglandin, and the main purpose is to enable blood flow to the penis, thereby creating an erection.

Trimix contains three agents: prostaglandin, papaverine and phentolamine. If Caverject does not work, then your urologist might go to the next line of treatment which is Trimix. Both injections must be injected in the right place, away from the urethra and main nerve on top of the penis, to be effective.

These injections are prescribed by either your urologist or urologist nurse practitioner, and a comprehensive education program is provided on the placement of the needle. You are also encouraged to practise how to inject yourself under the supervision of the doctor or a nurse.

In case you have injection phobia, you might get your wife or partner to administer the drug, and hopefully it does work as expected.

The penis injections are a combination of three medications and cannot be bought directly from the pharmacy. They are called 'compound medications' where a pharmacist makes them up according to the required combination of drugs, and prescription is required to access this injection. Furthermore, they are not cheap; an ongoing commitment of funds is required to purchase them.

It sounds easy, but it can sometimes take time to get the right dose; and sometimes it can be a total failure and does not achieve anything. Since with normal intimacy sex is spontaneous, the use of these injections can be off-putting due to the titrating needed to get the right dose. Therefore, it might take quite a long time to get the right dosage, if it works at all.

Intimacy is about feeling relaxed and spontaneous, so this process of requiring an injection and waiting for it to work can create a bit of stress and tension between couples. The loss of spontaneity makes intimacy more mechanical and less enjoyable for some. It takes patience, the understanding of your partner, perseverance and working as a team if success is to be achieved.

The whole process can also take away the enthusiasm for couples, so one or the other may end up feeling let down or lacking the urge for intimacy. So sexual satisfaction for both partners can be difficult.

Therefore, while support like injections is available to aid you in achieving penetrative sex, the process can be overwhelming in terms of your mental wellbeing.

Some men are lucky enough to get the functional dose right straight away and hence their sex lives are restored. Those who do not achieve the optimal results with the injections might keep on trying to titrate, or give up all together after a few attempts.

Advantages of Using Trimix Injections

The benefits of Trimix are:-

- Works 10 to 15 minutes after administration
- 90% effective
- It is safe and reliable
- Not affected by alcohol consumption.

As with every other drug there are side effects associated with the administration of Trimix, such as stinging at the injection site.

An erection of more than four hours after administration is a medical emergency and you should present yourself at the hospital. There is an antidote to this injection, but if it's taken and the erection is still persistent then there is no other choice but to go to the hospital for treatment.

Men think it is embarrassing going to the hospital with an erection. However, given the pain associated with this for a long time, shame is irrelevant. You need to understand that doctors see these kinds of cases all the time and they never judge patients presenting with this issue.

Disadvantages of Trimix

As with all medical interventions, not all these medications perform as required. With Trimix there are some men for whom the injection might not work, irrespective of the dosage. In this case, men can try the strongest dose and it still might not work on their body.

The cause of this may be venous leakage, arterial inefficiency or another medical condition as mentioned above.

Where Trimix injections have failed, it is possible that a penile implant could be recommended. Again, have these discussions with your urologists and investigate the best options for your individual case.

Peyronie's Disease

After using Caverject and Trimix over a long period of time, 15 to 20% of men develop signs of Peyronie's disease. This is due to repeated injections on the penis, which create scar tissue. It can present itself as a lump, curvature, penile shortening or hourglass (narrowing) appearance. You would be alarmed if you saw your penis changing shape, so seek help.

Men who use penile injections are prone to developing Peyronie's disease because the penile tissue does not have enough blood flow and therefore it can take a long time for the tissues to repair themselves.

Treatments for Peyronie's disease include surveillance, penile traction, or direct injection on the penis to try and treat the condition, with surgery as a last resort.

Penile Implant

Penile implants are prosthetic devices inserted in your penis that facilitate achieving an erection for penetrative sexual satisfaction. The implants come in different types and therefore it is important to undertake full research on the benefits and disadvantages of each type of prosthesis.

Penile implants are the last resort for treating erectile dysfunction if all other interventions fail to achieve the intended results. Research shows that 80% of men who have undergone penile implant have satisfying results.

There are three types of penile implants, namely:

- Malleable or semi-rigid rods - They comprise of two flexible rods inserted on each side of the penis.

These rods never change in size or stiffness and maintain semi-rigid state. They can be bent downwards as well as upwards for sexual activity. However, due to their flexibility they can be uncomfortable and not easy to hide under one's clothing.

- Two-piece inflatable implants - These come as inflatable cylinders which are inserted inside the shaft of the penis while a fluid reservoir and pump is placed in the scrotum. The cylinders do not fully deflate.

- Three-piece implant - This is the most common form of penile implant, with a good reported success rate. It consists of three components: two cylinders, a pump and a reservoir. The cylinders are inserted into the penis, the pump in the scrotum and the reservoir in the abdomen. This implant creates a rigid erection by means of pumping on the pump, which inflates the cylinders. On releasing the pump, the cylinders deflate, and this returns the penis to a flaccid state.

While penile implants provide a satisfactory outcome, for some men there can be side effects. Mechanical faults can be one of them, where the implant does not work, requiring a new one to be inserted. Since this is a surgical procedure which requires incision on your body, infection can occur, and this can affect the healing process and create discomfort.

It is also important to ensure that you communicate with your doctor concerning any previous procedures undertaken on your abdomen, so as the surgeon can avoid any areas where scar tissue is present. For example, some men may have had hernia repair undertaken and mesh put in place to avoid hernia recurrence.

Other considerations for suitability apply to men who suffer from cardiovascular disease and diabetes, since medications for these conditions might need to be assessed before any surgical procedure is undertaken. The more information you provide to your surgeon the better the outcome.

Open Communication Strategy

Open communication is important in relationships, and some couples find it comfortable to talk about everything in their lives – except the area of sexual health. It can be difficult to initiate such discussions if you have been in a relationship for a long time but have never talked about your sexual life.

However, once the disease strikes, such discussions can be difficult to avoid. Nevertheless, there are those who find this area of discussion confronting and are uncomfortable being intimate in this way. They tend to avoid talking about these sensitive issues altogether.

There is no shame in discussing the issues associated with prostate with your wife and or partner, since you care and value them as part of your family. Even when men have a tendency to brush it off, women can initiate the discussion about what happens after treatment, and how both partners can tackle the challenges associated with the side effects.

If discussion of this topic proves difficult, counselling from a sexual health professional who deals with prostate issues would be an ideal next move. When communication doors remain shut, your partner could become very frustrated with tackling this prostate journey, and they might not have anybody to turn to for advice or support.

Over the years I have realised that this disease can slowly estrange couples, even when they have been together for many years. At times, men can suffer from related mental health issues, or can feel frustrated by not being able to provide an intimate relationship for their partners. At this point, otherwise strong relationships sometimes break down, and people go their own separate ways.

Some men are also filled with anger associated with being 'deprived of their manhood' The societal perception of what a man 'should' be, and the mental anguish associated with this, can create a very hostile environment if the man feels he is 'not man enough'.

In this case open communication, and perhaps counselling, can play a great role in reassuring him that it is not sexual activity alone that makes one a man. There are other ways t o express love, by caring for one another, closeness and cuddling, and playing with one another. Taking things one step at a time is the ideal path to follow.

Remission and Raising of PSA

The whole point of having prostate treatment, whether invasive or not, is to ensure that cancer is under control and is in remission. Some people are lucky -- they manage to have their cancers under control -- while others are not so lucky, and experience a recurrence. This can happen when cancers are very aggressive.

After completion of the initial treatment, and feeling like your life is under control, a continuous monitoring is undertaken over six and twelve months, depending on the results and your treating doctor.

Some people might not see an increase in PSA for a long time, but others are not so lucky. An alternative treatment is offered to ensure that PSA is controlled, and that cancer has not metastasised – that is, invaded other body parts, such as the lymph nodes and bones.

Palliative Care

There are a lot of myths associated with palliative care. Some people think that once you are under palliative care you are entering the last days of your life. People can literally view palliative care as the end-of-life place where only those awaiting to depart from this world are catered for.

While this can be true for some, it does not however mean that everybody who is under palliative care is nearing death. There are people who have been managed under palliative care and have lived well for long periods.

Therefore, you should not shy away from getting support from palliative care just because it is associated with dying people.

When cancer has grown to distant tissues and body systems, such as lymph nodes, other organs and the bones, the doctors might suggest a low dose maintenance medication to keep you comfortable and to improve quality of life where pain is well managed.

Radiation might also be an option, and in this case, it is not suggested as a cure but as a way of minimising pain, again providing you with comfort and quality of life.

All these options could be discussed with your treating doctor, who will suggest the best way possible to manage you. It is also your right to ask questions and to understand what the new treatment entails. Since prostate cancer, or any other disease, affects other family members too, it is important for them to be involved in your care so that everyone is on the same page.

Palliative care team work with a multidisciplinary team, analyses your individual case and provide support for your needs such as physical, emotional, psychological, financial and/or spiritual assistance. If any support could provide you with a comforatable life, why not embrace the opportunity and make use of it?

Finally, patients can feel that they might not be with their families for long, and that their health is not getting better; therefore, spending quality time with other family members at this stage would be beneficial to all. Putting your affairs in order can relieve family pressures too, so that when you are no longer there, the family does not have to worry about your estate.

This does not mean that being organised and writing up a will is a sign of death. However, it does eliminate a lot of problems if you are not around to sort things out. The last thing your family members would want after going through a distressing illness journey is to deal with unnecessary bureaucracy.

I am not a lawyer and not in any position to advise anyone on what they could do; however, having worked in hospitals for a long time, I have seen some unfortunately Distressing and avoidable situations.
Do prepare.

Conclusion

Prostate issues, including cancers, involve everyone in the family; therefore, they are not individual issues. They need to be seen primarily as a 'couple's disease', with an acknowledgement that other members of the family are involved. It is therefore important to include your wife and or partner when dealing with your prostate issues, as they will inevitably be affected in one way or another.

Walking together as a team on the journey to live with prostate problems can minimise a lot of family issues. You get the required support without feeling as if you are a burden to your partner, wife or family. The journey can be long and tedious, but collectively, you can achieve the goal of living a normal life, as dictated by your health.

Hopefully the medical profession will keep on improving and advancing prostate treatments to achieve much better outcomes for all.

References

Chung E. (2017). Penile prosthesis implant: scientific advances and technological innovations over the last four decades. Transl Androl Urol. 2017 Feb;6(1):37-45. doi: 10.21037/tau.2016.12.06. PMID: 28217449; PMCID: PMC5313299.

Pacik, Dalibor & Fedorko, Michal. (2017). Literature review of factors affecting continence after radical prostatectomy. Saudi Medical Journal. 38. 9-17. 10.15537/smj.2017.1.15293.

Scott, A.F.; Mohr, D.W.; Ling, H.; Scharpf, R.B.; Zhang, P.; Liptak, G.S.(2014) Characterization of the Genomic Architecture and Mutational Spectrum of a Small Cell Prostate Carcinoma.366-384.https:// doi.org/10.3390/genes5020366.

Xiang, J., Yan, H., Li, J. *et al (2019)* Transperineal versus transrectal prostate biopsy in the diagnosis of prostate cancer: a systematic review and meta-analysis. *World JSurg Onc* **17**, 31 (2019). https://doi.org/10.1186/s12957-019-1573-